KNOWLEDGE GUIDE TO
GOUT

Essential Manual To Symptoms, Treatments, Diets, And Natural Remedies For Lasting Relief

DR. AARON BRANUM

Copyright © 2024 BY DR. AARON BRANUM

All rights reserved. Except for brief quotations embodied in critical reviews and certain other noncommercial uses permitted by copyright law, no part of this publication may be reproduced, distributed, or transmitted in any form or by any means, Including photocopying, recording, or other electronic or mechanical methods, without the prior written permission of the publisher.

Disclaimer:

The data in this book, is solely meant to be informative and instructional.

This book is not intended to replace expert medical advice, diagnosis, or care. No medical, health, or other professional services are offered by the author, publisher, or any affiliated parties

Individual outcomes may differ in the practice of these therapies, which entail a variety of approaches and methodologies.

A one-on-one session with a trained or certified healthcare professional is still preferable. It is best to consult a trained healthcare provider before making any decisions regarding your health.

The author of this book is not affiliated with any specific website, product, or organization related to any of these therapies.

All reasonable measures have been taken by the author and publisher to guarantee the authenticity and dependability of the material contained in this book

Contents

CHAPTER ONE 15

GOUT UNDERSTANDING: WHAT IS IT AND WHY IS IT IMPORTANT? 15

- Gout Definition 15
- Reasons And Danger Elements 16
- Signs & Symptoms To Keep An Eye On 16
- The Value Of Early Identification And Treatment 17
- Effects On Everyday Life 18

CHAPTER TWO 21

GOUT'S HISTORY: CHATHING ITS ORIGINATION AND EVOLUTION 21

- A Historical View Of Gout 21
- Treatment And Understanding Evolution ... 22
- Cultural Myths And Perceptions Regarding Gout 22
- Famous People In The Gout History 23
- Perspectives Obtained From Past Cases 24

CHAPTER THREE 25

GOUT AND YOUR BODY: THE IMPACT ON YOUR WELL-BEING 25

  Comprehending Uric Acid And Its Function: 25

  Effects Of Gout On Mobility And Joints: 26

  Relationship Between Gout And Other Medical Disorders: 28

  Effects Over Time On General Health: 29

  The Value Of Comprehensive Management 31

CHAPTER FOUR 35

GOUT DIAGNOSIS: ACTIONS TO RECOGNISE AND VERIFY THE ILLNESS 35

  Symptoms And Indications To Watch Out For 35

  Diagnostic Procedures And Tests 36

  Diagnosis Differential From Other Conditions 38

  The Importance Of Physical Examination And Medical History 39

  Timely Diagnosis Is Essential For Effective Management 41

CHAPTER FIVE 43

OPTIONS FOR TREATMENT: FROM MEDICATION TO CHANGES IN LIFESTYLE ... 43

An Overview Of Available Medication 43

Diet And Nutrition's Role In Gout Management 47

The Significance Of Hydration And Lifestyle Adjustments 50

Complementary Methods And Alternative Therapies 52

Customized Plans Of Care And Things To Take Into Account 55

CHAPTER SIX 59

MANAGEMENT STRATEGIES FOR THE LONG TERM: PREVENTING GOUT FLARES 59

Recognizing Gout Flare Triggers 59

The Value Of Following Treatment Plans ... 61

Changes In Lifestyle To Avoid Flares 64

The Function Of Drugs In Preventing Flares 67

Keeping An Eye On And Modifying Management Strategies 69

CHAPTER SEVEN 73
MANAGEMENT AND COPING TIPS FOR DAILY LIVING WITH GOUT 73
Recognizing Your Symptoms And Triggers 73
Controlling Pain During Episodes 75
Coping Strategies For Mental Health 76
Long-Term Care Planning And Self-Advocacy 78

CHAPTER EIGHT 81
GOUT AND YOUR DIET: SELECTING FOODS TO IMPROVE YOUR HEALTH 81
Recognizing How Diet Affects Gout 81
Foods To Include And Foods To Avoid 81
The Significance Of Moderation And Portion Control 83
Techniques For Eating Out And Social Events 84
Consulting Healthcare Experts For Advice .85

CHAPTER NINE 87
GOING AHEAD: DIRECTING OUR ENERGY FUTURE 87
Long-Term Prognosis For Gout Patients 87

The Value Of Continued Monitoring And Aftercare 88
Possibilities For Raising Awareness And Advocacy 89
Promising Developments And Advancements In Research... 90
Giving People The Tools To Take Charge Of Their Health Journey 91

CONCERNING THIS BOOK

In the field of health literature, "Knowledge Guide to Gout" is a shining example of enlightenment, providing a thorough examination of the various facets of this sometimes misdiagnosed illness. The book delves into the complexities of gout, starting with the basics and giving readers a complete grasp of its definition, causes, and symptoms.

This explanation emphasizes the critical role awareness plays in reducing the impact on day-to-day living by providing readers with the knowledge necessary for early detection and proactive management.

The historical journey undertaken in this book provides an incisive analysis of cultural attitudes and myths surrounding the condition in addition to providing a retrospective look at the development of gout therapies.

Readers are given a wider knowledge of the relevance of the disease beyond its clinical signs by learning about its historical roots and the experiences of prominent persons. This historical contextualization attests to the fact that gout has remained relevant throughout history.

"Knowledge Guide to Gout" goes beyond historical accounts to clarify the complex relationship between gout and general health. The book highlights the connection between gout and other medical disorders by explaining the function of uric acid and how it affects joints and mobility.

This emphasizes the need for comprehensive therapeutic approaches. Readers are provided with essential insights on the long-term impacts of gout on their well-being through this holistic perspective, which empowers them to take proactive measures to protect their health.

The path to diagnosis that is explained in the pages of this book provides guidance for those who are struggling with the uncertainty around gout.

The diagnostic process is made clear to readers by outlining the signs and symptoms, tests, and medical history factors.

This gives them the ability to confidently and clearly negotiate this confusing terrain. People can regain control over their health journey by starting on a path of healing and restoration with prompt diagnosis and efficient care.

The therapeutic arsenal included in the book includes a variety of approaches, from drugs to way-of-life adjustments.

In order to help readers achieve maximum health, the book provides a comprehensive analysis of customized treatment programs and complementary therapies.

In addition, the focus on prevention highlights the proactive approach taken throughout the book, stressing the significance of following treatment regimens and making lifestyle changes to avoid flare-ups of gout.

"Knowledge Guide to Gout" acts as a culinary compass in the area of dietary issues, guiding readers prudently and wisely through the maze of food options.

By clarifying how nutrition affects gout and providing useful tips for handling social situations, the author gives readers the knowledge and resources they need to make decisions that support their health and vitality.

By means of this culinary enlightenment, people can set out on a path to holistic health, moving past the limitations of gout to welcome a future full of life and plenty.

CHAPTER ONE

GOUT UNDERSTANDING: WHAT IS IT AND WHY IS IT IMPORTANT?

Gout Definition

The accumulation of uric acid crystals in the joints causes gout, a complicated and excruciating ailment that is sometimes referred to as a kind of arthritis.

An overabundance of uric acid in the blood can cause these crystals to grow, which can cause excruciating pain, swelling, and inflammation. The big toe is typically affected, but it can also affect other joints such as the ankles, knees, wrists, and fingers.

Even the smallest movement can be unpleasant due to the agonizing pain, which is frequently described as abrupt and strong.

Reasons And Danger Elements

The condition known as hyperuricemia, which is characterized by an increased quantity of uric acid in the bloodstream, is one of the main causes of gout. Genetics, diets strong in purines (compounds found in foods like red meat, shellfish, and alcohol), obesity, high blood pressure, and certain drugs are some of the causes of this. In addition, those who have a family history of gout are more likely to get the illness themselves.

Signs & Symptoms To Keep An Eye On

Early intervention and therapy of gout depend on the ability to recognize its signs. Intense joint pain, which typically flares up unexpectedly and usually occurs at night or in the early morning, is the primary symptom.

The afflicted joint gets red, swollen, and incredibly sensitive to touch. Fever or chills might also be experienced by some individuals during a gout episode.

Differentiating gout from other joint-related illnesses, like infection or injury, is crucial because early treatment can reduce symptoms and avoid consequences.

The Value Of Early Identification And Treatment

Proactive management and early identification are essential for managing gout effectively and reducing its impact on day-to-day activities. Gout can cause joint injury, recurring flare-ups, and tophi (lumpy uric acid crystals under the skin) if treatment is not received.

In addition, uric acid accumulation in gout patients increases their risk of problems such as kidney stones and renal damage.

Thus, it is essential to seek medical assistance as soon as gout symptoms appear in order to ensure an accurate diagnosis and appropriate treatment planning.

Effects On Everyday Life

A person's quality of life can be greatly impacted by gout, which can make it difficult for them to carry out everyday chores and engage in enjoyable activities.

Gout episodes can render afflicted joints immobile due to the intense pain and swelling , making it intolerable to walk, stand, or even wear shoes.

The emotional toll of the illness can also be increased by worry and sadness brought on by the fear of suffering through another excruciating flare-up.

Effective gout management can minimize its negative effects on everyday activities and general well-being, help people reclaim control over their lives, and involve medication, lifestyle changes, and routine follow-ups with healthcare experts.

CHAPTER TWO

GOUT'S HISTORY: CHATHING ITS ORIGINATION AND EVOLUTION

A Historical View Of Gout

The history of gout, sometimes referred to as the "disease of kings" or "rich man's disease," is extensive and spans many centuries.

Ancient societies including the Greeks, Romans, and Egyptians identified and recorded this illness, linking it to lifestyle and food excesses. The Egyptian physician Imhotep's writings from 2600 BCE contain the earliest known references to gout. Gout has historically been linked to excess, overindulgence in rich meals, and a sedentary lifestyle, frequently affecting the wealthy and powerful.

Treatment And Understanding Evolution

Gout remedies have changed dramatically over the ages. Herbal medicines, bloodletting, and food restrictions were the mainstays of early treatment practices.

Gout was regarded as an excess disorder throughout the Middle Ages, and severe treatments like fasting and purging were frequently used to cure it.

The discovery of uric acid's significance in gout did not occur until the 18th century, which paved the way for the creation of more specialized treatments.

Cultural Myths And Perceptions Regarding Gout

Cultural misconceptions and beliefs about gout have persisted for a long time. It was seen as the result of moral failings and overindulgence in many countries. Class divisions and social hierarchies were strengthened as a result of the stigmatization of gout sufferers due to its link with excess and luxury. Misconceptions still exist today; some people think that dietary carelessness is the only cause of gout instead of underlying metabolic issues.

Famous People In The Gout History

Gout's status as a sickness of affluence has been cemented by the fact that many famous people throughout history have suffered from it. Among them are well-known kings, such as Louis XIV of France and Henry VIII of England, the latter of whom is well-known for his gout struggles in his final years. Gout is thought to have affected anyone, even well-known artists like Michelangelo and Leonardo da Vinci. This highlights how indiscriminate illness can be.

Perspectives Obtained From Past Cases

Examining past occurrences of gout offers important information regarding the disease's epidemiology, course, and social effects.

Researchers can learn about the frequency of gout in various historical times, its many forms, and the efficacy of therapies by looking through medical records, firsthand stories, and artistic renderings.

Furthermore, examining the gout-related experiences of historical personalities provides insight into societal and cultural perceptions of the illness and its treatment.

CHAPTER THREE

GOUT AND YOUR BODY: THE IMPACT ON YOUR WELL-BEING

Comprehending Uric Acid And Its Function:

The kidneys normally filter out uric acid, a result of purine biosynthesis, and eliminate it through urine. Gout, however, is caused by uric acid crystallizing and depositing in joints when levels of the substance are too high or the kidneys are unable to remove it effectively. It is essential to comprehend this process in order to appropriately manage gout.

Uric acid levels rise in gout patients, which causes needle-like crystals to grow in the joints, especially the big toe, ankles, knees, and wrists. These crystals cause severe inflammation and discomfort, which are frequently described as crippling and agonizing. It is essential to comprehend how uric acid accumulates and crystallizes in order to avoid and treat gout attacks.

It's also critical to identify the causes that lead to elevated levels of uric acid. Some foods high in purines, alcohol use, dehydration, obesity, and some drugs are examples of these triggers. People can lower their risk of gout flare-ups by adopting more educated lifestyle choices by being aware of these factors.

Effects Of Gout On Mobility And Joints:

Gout can have an adverse effect on several joints at once, greatly reducing the range of motion and general quality of life. Uric acid crystal inflammation can result in swelling, redness, warmth, and excruciating pain in the afflicted joints. Even small movements may become unbearable due to this discomfort, which is frequently described as throbbing.

Repeated bouts of gout can damage and deform joints over time, eventually resulting in chronic arthritis. If treatment is not received, this may further restrict mobility and raise the likelihood of impairment. Knowing how gout progresses and how it affects joints emphasizes the value of early intervention and proactive management techniques.

Gout can, in extreme circumstances, damage organs and tissues in addition to joints. As an illustration of the systemic nature of this disorder and the necessity for comprehensive therapy strategies, the accumulation of uric acid crystals in the kidneys can result in kidney stones or even damage to the kidneys.

Relationship Between Gout And Other Medical Disorders:

Gout is not a standalone ailment; it frequently coexists with other medical problems to create a complicated web of related disorders. Gout and metabolic syndrome, a group of illnesses that includes obesity, high blood pressure, insulin resistance, and dyslipidemia, are significantly correlated. Heart disease and other problems are more likely to occur when these disorders worsen one another.

Furthermore, gout is strongly associated with lifestyle choices including food and alcohol intake. Red meat, shellfish, and sugar-filled drinks are examples of foods high in purines that can raise uric acid levels and cause gout attacks. Additionally, alcohol—especially beer and spirits—can increase uric acid levels and exacerbate the symptoms of gout.

Comprehending these associations enables individuals to make knowledgeable decisions for better disease management.

Gout has also been linked to a higher chance of developing diabetes, hypertension, and chronic renal disease, among other illnesses. This emphasizes the significance of comprehensive management plans that deal with gout's underlying risk factors and associated medical disorders in addition to the disease itself.

Effects Over Time On General Health:

Even though gout attacks might appear to be isolated bouts of discomfort and inflammation, if the condition is not treated, it can have a major long-term impact on general health. Gout-related chronic inflammation has been connected to a higher risk of cardiovascular illness, which includes heart attacks and strokes.

In addition, long-term elevated uric acid levels may be linked to kidney stones and chronic renal disease, which eventually results in a progressive loss of kidney function. These side effects highlight how crucial it is to control uric acid levels, address underlying risk factors, and treat acute gout attacks in order to avoid long-term health effects.

Gout also has an impact on one's quality of life and mental health in addition to physical health. Anxiety, despair, and a decline in social functioning are among the mental health consequences that can result from long-term pain, incapacity, and the unpredictable nature of gout attacks. To improve overall health outcomes and enable complete care of gout, it is imperative to acknowledge and address these psychosocial elements of the disease.

The Value Of Comprehensive Management

Effective gout management necessitates a thorough, multidimensional strategy that takes into account underlying risk factors, associated medical disorders, and acute symptoms.

To attain the best results, this all-encompassing management approach includes pharmacological therapy, lifestyle changes, and routine monitoring.

Dietary modifications are essential for managing gout; purine-rich food reduction, moderation in alcohol use, and maintenance of a healthy weight are prioritized. Frequent exercise can help lower uric acid levels, lessen inflammation, and increase joint mobility.

Preventing dehydration and remaining hydrated is also crucial in order to avoid gout attacks.

In order to reduce uric acid levels and stop flare-ups in the future, medication therapy might be required.

This may involve drugs like probenecid, febuxostat, or allopurinol that either increase or decrease the excretion of uric acid. To determine the safest and most successful treatment plan that is customized to each patient's needs, close collaboration with a healthcare professional is vital.

It is crucial to regularly monitor uric acid levels and general health in order to evaluate the effectiveness of treatment and make any necessary adjustments. Periodic blood tests, joint checks, and consultations with healthcare specialists are possible measures to guarantee the best possible care and avoid any issues.

Because gout is a complicated ailment, therapy must be approached from all angles. People with gout can enhance their quality of life and effectively manage their illness by being aware of the function that uric acid plays, the effects it has on joints and general health, and the links it has with other medical conditions.

CHAPTER FOUR

GOUT DIAGNOSIS: ACTIONS TO RECOGNISE AND VERIFY THE ILLNESS

Symptoms And Indications To Watch Out For

Often called the "disease of kings" or "rich man's disease," gout is a kind of arthritis brought on by an accumulation of crystals made of uric acid in the joints. Understanding the telltale signs and symptoms of gout is essential for prompt diagnosis and efficient treatment.

Abrupt and severe joint pain, usually in the big toe but also affecting other joints, is the classic sign of gout. This pain is usually sudden, usually occurs at night, and may be accompanied by warmth, redness, and swelling in the afflicted joint. Other typical symptoms include restricted joint range of motion and persistent soreness that persists long after the initial pain goes away.

In addition to joint pain, fever, and chills are examples of systemic symptoms that can accompany acute flare-ups of gout. These symptoms are very important to monitor, particularly if they worsen or return over time, as they may be signs of underlying gout.

Diagnostic Procedures And Tests

A combination of laboratory testing and clinical assessment is used to diagnose gout. A complete medical history and physical examination might yield important hints, but laboratory confirmation is frequently needed for a final diagnosis. Joint fluid analysis is one of the most often utilized tests; it involves taking a tiny sample of fluid from the afflicted joint and looking for urine crystals under a microscope. Gout is characterized by these needle-like crystals that exhibit negative birefringence when viewed under polarised light.

Through the measurement of uric acid levels in the bloodstream, blood tests can also assist in the diagnosis of gout.

It's crucial to remember that raised uric acid levels by themselves do not guarantee a diagnosis of gout, as many people with hyperuricemia—high uric acid levels—do not experience gout and other gout sufferers may experience severe flare-ups with normal uric acid levels.

Over time, imaging techniques like dual-energy CT scans, ultrasounds, and X-rays can be useful in determining the extent of joint damage caused by gout.

Characteristic results that may not be visible with a physical examination alone, like urate deposits (tophi) and joint degradation, can be found with these tests.

Diagnosis Differential From Other Conditions

Since gout can mimic other types of arthritis and inflammatory diseases, a precise diagnosis is crucial to prevent mishandling the situation. Pseudogout is a disorder that resembles gout in that it is brought on by the buildup of calcium pyrophosphate crystals in the joints.

Although the two disorders can be distinguished from one another despite the similarity in their clinical manifestation, pseudogout can be distinguished from gout due to the differences in the crystals involved and how they appear under a microscope.

The differential diagnosis should also take into account other illnesses such as rheumatoid arthritis, osteoarthritis, and septic arthritis that may manifest as joint pain and swelling. Gout can be distinguished from these other disorders with the use of a comprehensive evaluation that includes a review of the patient's medical history, a physical examination, and relevant diagnostic tests.

The Importance Of Physical Examination And Medical History

Since certain factors raise the chance of having gout, a thorough medical history is essential for the diagnosis of the ailment.

These include obesity, a high purine-rich food diet (red meat and shellfish), a high alcohol intake, a family history of gout, certain drugs (aspirin and diuretics), and underlying medical disorders (hypertension, diabetes, kidney disease).

Healthcare professionals will check for edema, redness, and warmth in the afflicted joint during the physical examination as indicators of inflammation.

In order to measure a range of motion and detect any discomfort, they might also palpate the joint.

They will also ask about the duration and frequency of symptoms, as well as any aggravating circumstances that could lead to flare-ups of gout.

Timely Diagnosis Is Essential For Effective Management

For the best results and to avoid complications, gout must be diagnosed as soon as possible. Urate deposits called tophi can accumulate in the soft tissues surrounding the joints as a result of untreated or improperly managed gout, which can also cause joint injury and frequent flare-ups. These issues raise the possibility of long-term incapacity and have a substantial negative influence on quality of life.

Furthermore, prompt identification enables the implementation of suitable treatment plans to lessen inflammation, lower blood levels of uric acid, and relieve symptoms. Changes in nutrition, weight loss, and alcohol intake can all help avoid flare-ups of gout and lower the chance of subsequent episodes. To treat acute flares and stop recurrence, doctors may also prescribe medications including colchicine, corticosteroids, nonsteroidal anti-inflammatory medicines (NSAIDs), and urate-lowering treatments (such as febuxostat and allopurinol).

Gout symptoms and indicators should be recognized as soon as possible, and a complete diagnostic examination is essential to determining the best course of treatment and enhancing patient outcomes.

Healthcare professionals can assist patients in properly managing their gout and lessen its impact on their everyday lives by diagnosing and treating the ailment as soon as possible.

CHAPTER FIVE

OPTIONS FOR TREATMENT: FROM MEDICATION TO CHANGES IN LIFESTYLE

An Overview Of Available Medication

Medication is a vital component of gout management since it helps to reduce symptoms and stop flare-ups in the future. Many kinds of drugs are available, and each one has a distinct function in the treatment of this illness.

Nonsteroidal Anti-Inflammatory Drugs (NSAIDs): During gout attacks, these medications are frequently used to lessen pain and inflammation. NSAIDs function by preventing the body from producing prostaglandins, which are chemicals that cause inflammation. Ibuprofen, naproxen, and indomethacin are a few examples.

Colchicine: Another drug that is often administered for gout is colchicine. It functions by lessening the pain and inflammation brought on by gout attacks.

Colchicine can be used as a prophylactic measure as well, but it works best when taken as soon as an attack is suspected.

Corticosteroids: Corticosteroids may be administered in situations where NSAIDs or colchicine are not appropriate or efficient. These drugs function by lowering inflammation and inhibiting the immune system's reaction to crystals of uric acid. Corticosteroids can be given intravenously, orally, or by injection into the afflicted joint.

Xanthine Oxidase Inhibitors, or XOIs, are a class of drugs that function by reducing the body's uric acid synthesis.

These drugs assist in reducing blood uric acid levels by blocking the xanthine oxidase enzyme, which is involved in the synthesis of uric acid. Febuxostat and allopurinol are two examples.

Uricosuric Agents: Uricosuric agents are drugs that cause the kidneys to excrete more uric acid, which lowers the blood levels of uric acid. XOIs and these drugs are frequently used to provide the best possible uric acid management. Lesinurad and probenecid are two examples.

Pegloticase: Pegloticase is an injectable biological drug that functions by changing uric acid into a more soluble form that the body can eliminate more readily.

Usually, it is saved for severe gout cases that have not improved with conventional therapies.

Biologics that reduce inflammation: These more recent drugs, such as IL-1 inhibitors, target particular inflammatory pathways linked to gout. When all other treatments have failed to control severe or refractory gout, they are frequently utilized.

Every drug option has advantages and possible drawbacks, and the choice of treatment will be influenced by a number of variables, including the patient's preferences, the severity of their gout, and the existence of any coexisting medical problems.

Diet And Nutrition's Role In Gout Management

Nutrition and diet are important in controlling gout and lowering the frequency of flare-ups. A person's risk of gout attacks may increase due to certain foods and beverages that raise blood levels of uric acid. On the other hand, altering one's diet can assist reduce uric acid levels and enhance the way gout is managed overall.

Eat Less Purine-Rich Foods: Purines are naturally occurring substances that can raise the body's uric acid levels. Red meat, organ meats, shellfish, and some fish varieties, such as sardines and anchovies, are foods high in purines. Reducing the amount of these foods consumed can help lower the chance of gout attacks.

Increased Intake of Low-Purine Foods: On the other hand, eating foods low in purines can help reduce uric acid levels and the frequency of flare-ups of gout. Nuts, legumes, whole grains, fruits, and vegetables are a few foods that are low in purines.

Keep Yourself Hydrated: Maintaining proper hydration is crucial for managing gout because it keeps uric acid from crystallizing in the joints. The risk of gout attacks can be decreased and excess uric acid can be flushed from the body by drinking lots of water throughout the day.

Limit Your Alcohol Consumption: Drinking alcohol, especially beer and spirits, can cause dehydration and raise the formation of uric acid, both of which can lead to gout attacks. Reducing the amount of alcohol consumed, particularly beer and spirits, can help lower the frequency of flare-ups related to gout.

Keep a Healthy Weight: Because obesity is linked to higher blood levels of uric acid, it increases the chance of developing gout. Combining diet and exercise to lose weight can help lower uric acid levels and reduce the incidence of gout attacks.

Think About Dietary Supplements: Research has indicated that certain dietary supplements, such as vitamin C and cherry extract, may help manage gout. Before adding supplements to your regimen, you should, however, speak with your healthcare provider about their use.

Gout sufferers can lessen the frequency of excruciating flare-ups and effectively manage their condition by changing their diet and forming good eating habits.

The Significance Of Hydration And Lifestyle Adjustments

Staying hydrated and making lifestyle changes are essential for controlling gout and preventing recurring attacks, in addition to medication and food adjustments. Including these routines in daily life can enhance the quality of life and facilitate the management of gout overall.

Keep Yourself Hydrated: Drinking enough water is crucial to removing excess uric acid from the body and avoiding uric acid crystallization in the joints. Try to consume eight glasses or more of water each day, especially when the weather is hot or you're exercising.

Keep a Healthy Weight: Because obesity is linked to greater blood levels of uric acid, it poses a serious risk for gout. Gout flare-up frequency can be decreased by achieving and maintaining a healthy weight with a balanced diet and frequent exercise.

Exercise Frequently: Frequent exercise helps lower blood levels of uric acid, minimize inflammation, and enhance joint function. Try to get in at least 150 minutes a week of moderate-to-intense exercise, including cycling, swimming, or brisk walking.

Handle Stress: Finding healthy methods to reduce stress and encourage relaxation is crucial because stress can aggravate symptoms of gout and cause attacks.

Deep breathing techniques, yoga, meditation, and time spent in nature are a few practices that can help lower stress and enhance general well-being.

Get Enough Sleep: Sleep deprivation raises the risk of gout attacks and inflammation. Aim for seven to nine hours of good sleep each night and follow good sleep hygiene practices, like sticking to a regular sleep schedule and establishing a calming bedtime ritual.

Gout sufferers can improve their general health and lessen the frequency and intensity of flare-ups by making drinking enough water a priority, establishing good lifestyle practices, and controlling their stress and sleep.

Complementary Methods And Alternative Therapies

Some gout sufferers may look into complementary and alternative therapies in addition to traditional medicine and lifestyle changes in order to control their symptoms and enhance their quality of life. Although these therapies might not be a replacement for medical care, they can be combined with traditional therapies to offer extra assistance.

Acupuncture: Acupuncture is a traditional Chinese medicine in which tiny needles are inserted into certain body sites to induce pain relief and healing. Acupuncture may help some gout sufferers reduce inflammation and relieve joint discomfort brought on by gout attacks.

Herbal medicines: For millennia, inflammatory diseases like gout have been treated with specific herbs and plant-based medicines. Turmeric, ginger, boswellia, and sour cherry extract are a few examples. Although there isn't much data on these gout cures' efficacy, some people could find them helpful when used in conjunction with more extensive treatment.

Massage Therapy: Massage therapy helps ease muscular tension, enhance blood flow, and lessen joint discomfort and inflammation. For those suffering flare-ups of gout, gentle massage techniques like Swedish or lymphatic drainage massage may be helpful.

Heat and Cold Therapy: Applying heat or cold to the afflicted joints might help ease pain and reduce inflammation during gout attacks. Heat therapy, such as warm compresses or heating pads, can assist relax muscles and enhance blood flow to the affected area. Cold therapy, such as ice packs or cold compresses, can numb the area and minimize swelling.

Dietary Supplements: In addition to vitamins and minerals, several dietary supplements may have anti-inflammatory qualities that can aid patients with gout. Examples include omega-3 fatty acids, vitamin D, and magnesium. But before taking any new supplements, it's crucial to speak with a healthcare professional to be sure they're safe and suitable for your particular requirements.

While some gout sufferers may find that complementary and alternative therapies help with their symptoms, it's important to proceed cautiously and speak with a healthcare professional to make sure they're safe and appropriate for your particular circumstances.

Customized Plans Of Care And Things To Take Into Account

Since each gout patient is different, their treatment strategy should be customized to meet their requirements, preferences, and medical background. A customized approach to managing gout considers a number of variables, such as the severity of the illness, the frequency of flare-ups, the existence of coexisting medical illnesses, and certain lifestyle choices.

Medical History: Creating a customized gout treatment plan requires a comprehensive evaluation of the patient's medical history. This includes determining whether any underlying illnesses, such as hypertension, diabetes, or kidney disease, may exacerbate gout or have an impact on available treatments.

The severity of Symptoms: Gout symptoms can range widely in intensity from little discomfort to severe pain and damage to joints. The intensity of the symptoms and the effect of gout on the patient's quality of life will determine the course of treatment.

Medication Tolerance and Preferences: Certain gout treatments may cause bad effects or contraindications for some people. When creating a treatment plan, it's critical to take the patient's medication tolerance and preferences into account. You should also collaborate with the patient to identify the most efficient and manageable solutions.

Lifestyle Factors: A person's diet, exercise routine, stress level, and alcohol intake can all have a big impact on how well they manage their gout. In addition to addressing these issues, a customized treatment plan will include advice on how to modify one's lifestyle for the better and promote overall gout control.

Follow-Up Care: To assess the efficacy of treatment and make any required modifications, routine follow-up visits with a healthcare professional are crucial. The doctor can evaluate gout symptoms, check uric acid levels, and offer continuing support and information for treating the condition during these visits.

Healthcare professionals may enhance treatment outcomes and raise the quality of life for gout sufferers by managing the ailment individually for each patient and taking into account their unique needs and preferences.

CHAPTER SIX

MANAGEMENT STRATEGIES FOR THE LONG TERM: PREVENTING GOUT FLARES

Recognizing Gout Flare Triggers

Many variables can cause gout flare-ups, and knowing what these triggers are is essential to managing the condition well.

Dietary choices, especially those heavy in purines such as red meat, seafood, and alcohol, are one of the main triggers.

These meals high in purines can raise the body's uric acid levels, which can cause urate crystals to develop in the joints and cause gout attacks.

Dehydration is another prevalent cause of flare-ups in gout. Uric acid can concentrate more in the bloodstream when the body is dehydrated, which raises the risk of crystal formation in the joints. Consequently, the key to avoiding gout flare-ups is to maintain proper hydration throughout the day by drinking lots of water.

As a side effect, some drugs can also cause flare-ups of gout. For instance, the body's uric acid levels might rise after using diuretics, which are frequently used to treat edema and high blood pressure.

Gout sufferers should talk to their doctor about their drug schedule in order to determine any possible triggers and, if necessary, look into other treatment alternatives.

In addition, lifestyle variables including stress, weight, and inactivity can exacerbate flare-ups of gout. Stress can make the body more inflammatory, and obesity and sedentary lifestyles are linked to greater uric acid levels and worse general health, which raises the likelihood of gout attacks.

Individuals suffering from gout can lessen the frequency and intensity of flare-ups by being aware of and able to detect these triggers. This could entail altering their food, drinking enough of water, controlling their stress levels, keeping a healthy weight, and talking to their doctor about possible prescription alternatives.

The Value Of Following Treatment Plans

Following treatment regimens is essential to controlling gout and lowering the chance of flare-ups. As gout is a chronic ailment that needs to be managed over time, following the recommended treatment plan is crucial to getting the best results.

Medication is one of the mainstays of gout treatment. This may involve pharmaceuticals like corticosteroids or nonsteroidal anti-inflammatory drugs (NSAIDs) to control pain and inflammation during flare-ups, as well as treatments like allopurinol or febuxostat to lower the body's uric acid levels. It is essential to take these drugs according to the recommended dosage and timing in order to manage symptoms and avoid more gout attacks.

A vital component of managing gout is making lifestyle changes in addition to taking medication. This can entail cutting back on purine-rich items in the diet, keeping a healthy weight, drinking enough of water, and exercising frequently. Following these lifestyle changes can help reduce uric acid levels, lessen the frequency of flare-ups of gout, and enhance general health.

Additionally, it's critical to regularly evaluate patients and follow up with healthcare practitioners to make sure treatment plans are operating as intended and to make any required modifications. This could entail routine blood work to check uric acid levels and continuing conversations about drug adherence and symptom management with medical professionals.

All things considered, following treatment regimens is essential to properly managing gout and lowering the likelihood of flare-ups. Gout sufferers can take charge of their health and have a higher quality of life by taking their prescription drugs as directed, changing their lifestyle, and staying in constant contact with their medical professionals.

Changes In Lifestyle To Avoid Flares

Changing one's lifestyle is essential to efficiently managing gout and preventing flare-ups. Gout sufferers can enhance their general quality of life and lessen the frequency and intensity of their attacks by changing to healthier behaviors.

Dietary adjustments are among the most significant lifestyle changes for reducing flare-ups of gout. Reducing your intake of purine-rich foods including red meat, organ meats, seafood, and alcohol can help lower your blood uric acid levels and lessen your chance of developing joint crystals. Those who have gout should instead concentrate on eating a well-balanced diet full of nutritious grains, fruits, vegetables, and lean meats.

Preventing flare-ups of gout also requires maintaining adequate hydration. By lowering the amount of uric acid in the blood and encouraging the kidneys to excrete it, drinking lots of water throughout the day helps control uric acid levels. Try to consume eight glasses of water or more each day, and avoid alcohol and sugar-filled drinks as these can also lead to dehydration.

Preserving a healthy weight is an additional crucial lifestyle adjustment to help avoid flare-ups of gout. Being obese increases inflammation and the body's uric acid levels, which makes it a major risk factor for gout. Reducing weight by means of a balanced diet and consistent exercise will help lower uric acid levels and lessen the frequency of gout attacks.

Apart from making dietary adjustments and controlling weight, consistent exercise helps avoid flare-ups of gout. Walking, swimming, or cycling are examples of low-impact exercises that can help increase joint mobility, lessen inflammation, and enhance general health. To see the advantages, try to get in at least 30 minutes of moderate-intensity activity most days of the week.

Gout sufferers can experience better long-term control of their ailment and a considerable reduction in the likelihood of flare-ups by implementing these lifestyle changes. Making these adjustments may require some time and work, but the advantages of better health and fewer gout symptoms make the effort worthwhile.

The Function Of Drugs In Preventing Flares

In order to effectively manage gout and avoid flare-ups, medications are essential. Gout can be treated with a variety of drugs, each having a special mode of action and advantages.

Urate-lowering treatment (ULT) is one of the main drug types used to treat gout. These drugs function by reducing the body's uric acid levels, which lessens the likelihood of gout flare-ups and helps stop urate crystals from forming in the joints. Probenecid, which enhances uric acid excretion through the kidneys, and allopurinol and febuxostat, which decrease the synthesis of uric acid, are often recommended ULT medicines.

There are drugs to control pain and inflammation during acute flare-ups of gout in addition to ULT medicines. Ibuprofen and naproxen are two examples of nonsteroidal anti-inflammatory medications (NSAIDs) that are frequently used to treat gout attacks by reducing inflammation and easing discomfort. During flare-ups, corticosteroids may also be administered to treat symptoms quickly.

An additional drug that can be used to treat and prevent gout flare-ups is colchicine. Colchicine helps relieve pain and swelling during flare-ups by lowering inflammation and blocking the migration of white blood cells to the afflicted joints. It can be used as a therapy option during acute flare-ups or as a prophylactic tactic to lessen the frequency of gout attacks.

The selection of a drug for the therapy of gout is contingent upon a number of aspects, such as the degree of symptoms, the existence of concomitant conditions, and the preferences of the individual patient.

Gout sufferers should collaborate closely with their physicians to create a customized treatment plan that takes into account their particular requirements and objectives.

Keeping An Eye On And Modifying Management Strategies

To properly control gout and prevent flare-ups, management tactics must be adjusted and monitored on a regular basis.

As gout is a chronic ailment, it needs to be continuously monitored, and the key to getting the best results is to be proactive in tracking the condition's symptoms and treatment effects.

Monitoring blood uric acid levels is one of the main ways to keep an eye on gout. In order to determine whether serum uric acid levels are within the target range for gout care, may entail routine blood testing.

By keeping an eye on uric acid levels, medical professionals can assess the efficacy of urate-lowering therapy (ULT) drugs and modify the dosage or course of treatment as needed.

People with gout should keep an eye on their symptoms and the frequency of their flare-ups in addition to their uric acid levels.

Maintaining a blog or diary of your gout attacks can be very helpful in identifying any patterns or triggers—such as dietary choices, alcohol consumption, or medication adherence—that may be causing flare-ups.

Making educated decisions on your course of treatment and lifestyle changes can be aided by this information.

Maintaining gout and modifying treatment plans as necessary also require routine follow-up visits with medical professionals.

Healthcare professionals can evaluate medication adherence, address any changes or concerns since the last visit, and evaluate gout symptoms during these appointments.

The treatment strategy may be modified in light of this information in order to maximize efficacy and reduce the chance of flare-ups.

All things considered, the key to successfully controlling gout and lowering the chance of flare-ups is proactive monitoring and modification of management techniques.

Gout sufferers can take charge of their health and have a higher quality of life by monitoring their uric acid levels, being aware of their symptoms, and communicating openly with medical professionals.

CHAPTER SEVEN

MANAGEMENT AND COPING TIPS FOR DAILY LIVING WITH GOUT

Gout necessitates a complex approach to everyday management and coping mechanisms. There are doable actions you can do to make life with this disease easier, even though it can be difficult at times.

Recognizing Your Symptoms And Triggers

Knowing your gout triggers and symptoms is one of the first steps in managing the condition. Maintain a notebook to record the meals, activities, and stressors that might trigger flare-ups. Certain purine-rich meals, such as red meat, seafood, and alcohol, are frequently identified as triggers. Finding trends will help you make decisions that will reduce the likelihood of flare-ups.

Optimal Eating Practices

Developing a balanced diet is essential to gout management. Prioritize eating a diet full of nutritious grains, fruits, vegetables, lean proteins, and balance. Eat fewer high-purine foods and avoid sugary drinks, as these might make gout symptoms worse. Drink lots of water to stay hydrated because dehydration can lead to flare-ups. Developing a customized meal plan with the assistance of a dietician can help you achieve your goals.

Adherence to Medication

Maintaining consistent medication compliance is crucial for managing gout symptoms and averting relapses. Even when you're feeling well, take your prescribed drugs as instructed by your healthcare practitioner. This could involve taking chronic drugs to lower blood levels of uric acid or drugs to lessen inflammation during flare-ups. If you have any side effects or questions concerning your drugs, consult your doctor.

Controlling Pain During Episodes

During flare-ups of gout, pain management is critical. Ibuprofen and naproxen, two nonsteroidal anti-inflammatory medications (NSAIDs), can help lessen pain and inflammation. Relief can also be obtained by applying ice packs to the injured joint. Pain can be reduced by resting and elevating the joint. For additional assessment and treatment options, speak with your healthcare physician if your pain continues or gets worse.

Including Exercise

Frequent exercise is good for your general health and can help control the symptoms of gout. Walking, swimming, and cycling are examples of low-impact workouts that are easy on the joints and can increase flexibility and mobility. On most days of the week, try to get in at least 30 minutes of moderate activity. As you feel comfortable, increase the intensity gently at first. Before beginning any new fitness regimen, make sure to speak with your healthcare physician.

Coping Strategies For Mental Health

Gout is one chronic ailment that can be very taxing on one's emotional health. Creating coping strategies is crucial if you want to control your stress and keep an optimistic attitude. Reduce stress by engaging in relaxation exercises like yoga, meditation, or deep breathing.

Take part in your favorite hobbies, like gardening, reading, or spending time with family and friends. Joining a support group or contacting a therapist can also be beneficial ways to get emotional assistance.

Creating a Network of Support

Creating a network of support is essential to successfully controlling gout. Assemble a support system of friends, family, and medical professionals who are aware of your situation and who can provide encouragement and support.

Joining an online forum or gout support group can help you meet people going through similar experiences.

You can feel less alone and more equipped to manage your illness by exchanging experiences and guidance with others.

Long-Term Care Planning And Self-Advocacy

Living with gout requires self-advocacy and long-term care planning. Create a thorough treatment plan that takes into account your unique requirements and objectives in collaboration with your medical team.

Take charge of your health by making an appointment for routine checkups, keeping an eye on your symptoms, and being honest with your healthcare practitioner.

Learn about gout and take charge of your own care and advocacy within the medical system.

Gout demands commitment, but with the correct techniques and assistance, you can successfully control your symptoms and enhance your quality of life.

You can take charge of your gout and lead a healthy life despite any difficulties it may cause by making healthy behaviors a priority, getting help, and standing up for yourself.

CHAPTER EIGHT

GOUT AND YOUR DIET: SELECTING FOODS TO IMPROVE YOUR HEALTH

Recognizing How Diet Affects Gout

One type of arthritis that is greatly influenced by diet is gout. The disorder develops as a result of uric acid crystals building up in the joints, which causes severe pain and inflammation.

The frequency and intensity of gout attacks can be greatly influenced by dietary choices, while heredity also plays a part.

Foods To Include And Foods To Avoid

Foods that either increase the body's production of uric acid or prevent it from being eliminated can cause flare-ups of gout.

Foods high in purines, such as organ meats, seafood, red meat, and sugar-filled drinks, are well-known offenders.

Because alcohol can increase uric acid levels, it's also important to limit alcohol consumption, especially beer and spirits.

Conversely, it may be advantageous to include meals that lower uric acid levels.

Cherries, for example, offer anti-inflammatory qualities that have been demonstrated to lessen gout attacks.

A gout-friendly diet can also contain whole grains, nuts, low-fat dairy products, and other fruits and vegetables.

The Significance Of Moderation And Portion Control

Controlling portion sizes is essential, even if some foods might not need to be completely avoided. If overindulged in, even healthful meals might aggravate gout.

Maintaining a healthy balance can be facilitated by keeping an eye on serving sizes and being aware of total calorie intake.

It is similarly crucial to exercise moderation when it comes to trigger foods. Even while it could be tempting to indulge sometimes, going beyond can have negative effects.

It's essential to learn to appreciate these meals in moderation if you want to effectively manage your gout.

Techniques For Eating Out And Social Events

For those with gout, navigating restaurant menus and social gatherings can be difficult. Nonetheless, it is easy to enjoy these times without aggravating symptoms with a little preparation and awareness.

When eating out, avoiding gout triggers can be achieved by choosing salads, vegetable-based dishes, grilled or baked lean meats, and seafood.

Requesting sauces and dressings separately helps you keep portions under control. Maintaining adequate hydration through water or unsweetened beverages can also help with the excretion of uric acid.

Informing the host of any dietary requirements or preferences can help to guarantee that appropriate options are provided when attending social occasions.

Additionally, you can ensure that there is something safe to eat by bringing gout-friendly food to share.

Consulting Healthcare Experts For Advice

Although dietary modifications are important in the management of gout, medical professionals should be consulted for specific advice.

Based on a patient's unique health requirements, prescription schedules, and lifestyle choices, a medical professional or registered dietitian can provide personalized guidance.

Scheduling routine check-ups with medical professionals enables continuous monitoring of gout symptoms and necessary dietary and treatment plan modifications.

Developing a cooperative relationship with a medical team is essential for better gout management through dietary and lifestyle changes.

CHAPTER NINE

GOING AHEAD: DIRECTING OUR ENERGY FUTURE

Gout is a journey towards long-term health management rather than merely a diagnosis. As vital as it is to address the symptoms right away, you need also to think about your overall health in the long run.

Long-Term Prognosis For Gout Patients

Recognizing that gout is a chronic ailment requiring continuing therapy is essential to understanding the long-term outlook for the condition. People suffering from gout can have happy, productive lives if they take proactive measures to reduce flare-ups and control their uric acid levels.

Changing one's diet, drinking plenty of water, keeping a healthy weight, and avoiding triggers like alcohol and particular foods are all part of managing gout. Long-term effectiveness also depends on frequent collaboration with medical specialists to check uric acid levels and modify medication as necessary.

The Value Of Continued Monitoring And Aftercare

Sustaining gout properly requires regular monitoring and follow-up care. This entails making appointments for routine check-ups with medical professionals to monitor uric acid levels, evaluate general health, and go over any modifications to symptoms or prescription requirements.

Healthcare providers can offer advice on medication adjustments, lifestyle changes, and ways to avoid flare-ups in the future during these consultations. Gout sufferers can enhance their overall quality of life and more effectively manage their condition by continuing to take an active and proactive role in their care.

Possibilities For Raising Awareness And Advocacy

Fighting myths and lowering the stigma associated with gout can be accomplished through advocacy and increased knowledge of the illness. People with gout can contribute to community efforts, support groups, and education by sharing personal experiences and encouraging empathy and understanding.

In addition, advocacy activities might concentrate on boosting funding for research, expanding access to healthcare resources, and supporting laws that assist gout sufferers. Patients, carers, medical professionals, and advocacy groups may all make a significant difference in the battle against gout by banding together.

Promising Developments And Advancements In Research

Improvements in gout diagnosis, care, and therapy are possible because of research advancements. Continued research is opening doors to better treatments and outcomes for gout sufferers, from novel drugs to fresh perspectives on the underlying causes of the illness.

Gout sufferers can actively contribute to the field's advancement and the development of future treatment choices by keeping up with the most recent research findings and, when suitable, taking part in clinical studies. Working together with researchers and healthcare professionals can also offer important chances to advance scientific understanding and influence gout treatment in the future.

Giving People The Tools To Take Charge Of Their Health Journey

The secret to effectively treating gout and preserving general health and well-being is empowerment. Gout sufferers who actively participate in their care are better able to make educated decisions, set reasonable objectives, and put self-management techniques into practice.

This could entail learning more about the illness, asking peers and medical professionals for help, and creating individualized plans for symptom management and flare-up prevention. Furthermore, engaging in self-care activities like relaxation, exercise, and stress reduction can enhance general health and quality of life.

By enabling gout patients to take charge of their own health care, we can build resilience, encourage self-sufficiency, and improve overall care satisfaction. Working together, we can create a day when people with gout are able to fully enjoy their lives without having to worry about their illness.

www.ingramcontent.com/pod-product-compliance
Lightning Source LLC
Chambersburg PA
CBHW071838210526
45479CB00001B/187